Electronic Cigarette

I0505751

The Ultimate Guide for Understanding E-Cigarettes and What You Need to Know

Recently, these three parts have been combined into one part, called the Cartomizer. And, as of late, an even more modernized form of the cartridge has been launched to the public, called the Clearomizer. "Re-buildable Atomizers" have also been introduced to the public recently.

Cartomizer

The Cartomizer is a form of e-liquid delivery system. It comprises a heating element inside of a poly-foam soaked in liquid. Also, you can dispose of it once you notice the liquid has a seemingly burnt taste. It is also important to note that cartomizers are mostly refillable.

Clearomizer

The Clearomizer uses a clear tank, in which the atomizer is inserted. There is no poly-foam material in Clearomizers and they use different wicking systems.

Re-buildable Atomizers

Re-buildable Atomizers allow users to assemble the wick, coil, and atomizers themselves.

Chapter 2:

Types of E-Cigarettes

Electronic cigarettes can be categorized into three distinct groups: **Cig-Alikes, Mid-Size, and Advanced Personal Vaporizers (APVs).** Here is what you need to know about them:

Cig-Alikes

Cig-Alikes are first generation electronic cigarettes that are popular because they look like real cigarettes, allowing smokers to feel comfortable. The only difference in size between Cig-Alikes and traditional cigarettes is that Cig-Alikes are normally heavier and bigger.

Cartomizers are great examples of Cig-Alikes. There are many flavors to choose from, and the most popular ones are Vanilla, Cherry, Menthol, Tobacco, and Lemon. There are also various nicotine levels to choose from, depending on your preference. You can choose from 0-24 grams of nicotine, or an even higher amount if you prefer.

Batteries can last up to several hours because they have a capacity range of 175 to 350 mAh. However, if you are looking to smoke a pack or more of Cig-Alikes in a day, then you definitely will need a spare battery with you.

There are also USB Cig-Alikes available. You can plug these into your computer or laptop and use them while working. Some of the most popular brands of Cig-Alikes are Eversmoke, Greensmoke, and South Beach Smoke. You can even use Eversmoke and South Beach Smoke with Greensmoke Batteries.

Mid-Size

Mid-Size are pen-shaped electronic cigarettes, also known as second-generation electronic cigarettes. Research shows Mid-Size electronic cigarettes are the most cost efficient of all the forms of electronic cigarettes. You can save up to 85% of smoking expenses if you use this form. Many cigarette users agree you will feel more fulfilled if you use the larger Mid-Size electronic cigarettes, because they can make you feel like you are using an actual cigarette. The batteries usually have a capacity of 350-1100 mAH and you need e-liquids for Mid-Size electronic cigarettes.

E-liquid is the solution used in electronic cigarette cartridges. There are three major components to e-liquids: Nicotine, Vaporizer, and Flavoring. Propylene Glycol is the most common of all e-liquid solutions. People with allergies or sensitivity to Propylene Glycol use Vegetable Glycerin as a substitution. A major advantage to using the Mid-Size electronic cigarette is that e-liquids can be mixed and matched, depending on one's preference.

Advanced Personal Vaporizers (APVs)

Advanced Personal Vaporizers, or APVs, are the most recently developed type of electronic cigarettes. They come in different shapes and sizes, from the simplest to the most unique. Some come in the form of gizmos or even screwdrivers. Electronic cigarette hobbyists and enthusiasts usually prefer this electronic cigarette, because it can be customized according to their tastes and preferences.

Advanced Personal Vaporizers require a large amount of e-liquid, so some non-hobbyists consider it very expensive. The good part about these though, is their batteries usually last longer, so you need not charge it repeatedly throughout the day.

You can also classify electronic cigarettes based on battery type. There are two types of batteries: **Automatic and Manual**

Automatic

An automatic battery type is one with an LED light on the end. This LED light automatically lights up when you inhale from the electronic cigarette.

Manual

A manual battery is one where you have to press the LED button and hold it while you inhale. While this may seem like more work initially, you will get used to it. Manual batteries give you more control over your vaping.

Lastly, electronic cigarettes can also be categorized based on their disposability and/or reusability. There are three categories:

Disposable Models

As the name suggests, you can dispose of these electronic cigarettes after use. This type is best for those who are curious about trying electronic cigarettes and are not looking to invest much money initially.

Disposable Cartomizers with Rechargeable Battery

The electronic cigarettes that fit into this category are mostly Cig-Alikes. If you do not like dealing with e-liquids or refilling, then this electronic cigarette is best for you.

Refillable Cartridges/Cartomizers with Rechargeable Battery

These are mostly the new electronic cigarettes, such as Mid-Size or pen style. You can recharge these batteries, refill these cartridges, and you will not have to buy e-liquid as often. Most electronic cigarette smokers choose this because of its reliability and they can use it repeatedly with less maintenance.

Now that you have an idea about the different electronic cigarettes and how they function, you can choose the electronic cigarette you think suits your budget and lifestyle. You can also try different electronic cigarettes at shops to see which one you like   best.

Chapter 3:

Positive Aspects

Some people have campaigned for the usage of electronic cigarettes over traditional tobacco cigarettes, and it is an ever-growing debate.

Here are the potential positive effects of using electronic cigarettes:

Using electronic cigarettes without nicotine alleviates the need to smoke. Also, it does not give smokers the usual withdrawal symptoms when they try to stop smoking, even for a night.

Even though nicotine concentration in the blood of smokers remains stable, their desire to quit smoking is still intact. So, sooner or later, the nicotine levels in their bodies will decline.

Electronic cigarettes reduce coughing in most individuals used to the heavy "smoker's cough", often associated with a cigarette addiction.

Because most people will buy a kit of starter cigarettes one time and can recharge the battery, electronic cigarettes allow consumers to save money. Instead of buying packs of traditional cigarettes daily, one would only need to buy a starter kit and then slowly buy e-liquids and pieces. This greatly reduces daily expenses and can help save money in the long run.

Electronic cigarette smokers also save others from health issues, due to reduced secondhand smoke. Secondhand smoke can cause certain illnesses, such as asthma, allergies, or even heart complications.

Because smoking traditional cigarettes has been known to cause bad breath, more people are inclined to use electronic cigarettes because they do not have the same effects. This is even more beneficial since there are many flavors that may help improve your breath, such as "mint" or "watermelon" flavored e-liquids.

Studies show that those who "vape" from electronic cigarettes have better palates than those who smoke traditional cigarettes. The vape smokers can taste and appreciate food better, because they do not taste burnt tobacco, and the taste of tobacco no longer overpowers the taste of real food.

It is also easier to get into better physical shape because your oxygen intake will no longer be blocked. Traditional cigarettes are full of carbon monoxide and therefore, block oxygen consumption in the body, which is bad for one's overall health.

There is an unfortunate stigma about smokers that they do not care about their image, appearance, or even the way they smell. By using electronic cigarettes, you can show the world you can do better and can smoke without hurting other people. Also, you can smell better, based on the flavors you choose.

Chapter 4:

Negative Aspects

As with most things in life, there are drawbacks and negative effects of using electronic cigarettes.

Here are some of the potential negative aspects to electronic cigarette use:

Some electronic cigarette users have said they have experienced symptoms of dehydration shortly after using their devices. This is most likely because the electronic cigarette contains propylene glycol, which has the ability to block water from circulating efficiently in the body. Some users have noticed they are allergic to propylene glycol, and this could be the reason for the reaction. Thorough research is still being done on this topic.

Despite best intentions, even kids and teenagers can buy electronic cigarettes, which is a disturbing idea. Because electronic cigarettes are more aesthetically pleasing than traditional cigarettes, teenagers and kids may feel tempted to buy them. Also, the fact that there are many delicious flavors could be a further source of temptation.

Although unlikely, there is still a possibility of nicotine overdose when one uses electronic cigarettes. Nicotine is proven to have negative effects in the control of blood sugar and in the circulation of blood throughout the body. Nicotine is also dangerous during pregnancy, whether inhaled by the smoker or passed on through secondhand smoke.

Other negative effects of nicotine include: emotional instability, mood swings, insomnia, and anxiety attacks. You may also experience extreme headaches, sweating, intestinal pain, coughing, a sore throat, and pain in your hands and feet. This is why it is important not to go all-out if you purchase an electronic cigarette. You need to make sure your body can handle all the possible effects of what you are inhaling.

One thing that potential electronic cigarette users fear the most is that the cigarette's battery may explode when over-charged or even while in normal use. As with any other battery-powered device, there is always a risk the battery may not work, become ruined, or even explode.

Another potential drawback to electronic cigarette users, by those who are used to smoking traditional cigarettes, can be the taste. Electronic cigarettes do not give that certain "edgy" taste and can be fruity or taste like menthol, depending on the quality of the e-liquid. Hardcore smokers do not really appreciate the flavor change, and sometimes, look down upon electronic cigarettes because of this. However, the quality of the electronic cigarette and the e-liquid being used can cause the experience to vary.

Unfortunately, electronic cigarettes may also cause pulmonary disorders in some people, just like traditional cigarettes. Those who do not know they are allergic to certain ingredients in electronic cigarette solutions may have coughing fits or asthma attacks, triggered by the inhalation of the solution.

Some electronic cigarette packs also lack certain regulatory factors, such as health warnings, a list of ingredients, mechanics on how to use them, and how to dispose of them properly. Because electronic cigarette makers are not asked to submit clinical data before producing electronic cigarette products, you can never be sure about the ingredients used, unless you do proper research into specific companies and products. This is why it is so important to go with well-known brands with solid reputations, rather than taking a risk with a low-quality product, just because it   is   cheaper.

Chapter 5:

More About Electronic Cigarettes

Typical electronic cigarette starter kits usually cost between $30 to $100. It is also common to find discounts and promotions on an electronic cigarette company website or in smoke shops. However, always be careful if you see an offer for a starter kit for an unusually low price. You do not want to gamble with a product you will use to inhale chemicals into your body, just because you want to save money on your purchase. Make sure the quality of any electronic cigarette you purchase is up to standards by thoroughly researching the manufacturing process of the product beforehand.

It is also worth noting that devices are uncontrolled and unregulated by the United States government; therefore, they are not banned in any areas. You can use electronic cigarettes in public places, without having to pay a fine or having to face legal charges. This is already changing, and laws can become different, so be informed of any new laws being enforced in your area regarding the usage of

While some electronic cigarettes are not rechargeable, such as the common ones found in gas stations or convenience stores, the majority of quality electronic cigarettes use rechargeable batteries that can last many months to a few years of regular use.

Cartridge

The cartridge is where the flavorings, nicotine, and liquid are contained. One cartridge usually is equivalent to around 250 puffs. However, more recent variations are expanding to higher numbers of puffs per cartridge. This amount of puffs per cartridge will probably increase in the next few years, as companies are trying to produce more efficient cartridges.

Despite all the changes and new innovations, electronic cigarettes still consist of three main parts: **an atomizer, a battery, and a cartridge.**

Atomizer

The atomizer is the central component of the electronic cigarette, alongside the battery. Atomizers handle the vaporization of the liquid. Atomizers can also be a wick material that draws in the liquid. Silica is also often used to make modern forms of the atomizer. However, other materials used to make atomizers include hemp, cotton, bamboo yam, steel mesh, and wire ropes.

Battery

The battery is used to give the electronic cigarette the power it needs to operate. They are mostly rechargeable and can allow the cigarette to be re-charged and used multiple times in a day, which is especially helpful if you are not fond of smoking a pack of cigarettes per day.

2007, and it is now the model used by major electronic cigarette companies. In the last few years, more companies are trying to come up with their own versions and variations of the electronic cigarette, and innovations are happening quicker than ever.

commercialized by 1967. The invention disappeared from the public eye, until the recent commercialization of the product.

Despite Mr. Gilbert's work, the form of the electronic cigarette widely used these days is credited to the invention in 2003, by a Chinese pharmacist named Hon Lik. This electronic cigarette used a piezoelectric-ultrasound element, similar to the electric charge accumulated in materials like ceramics, crystals, and even the human bone and DNA. This vaporizes a pressurized liquid jet of nicotine, which is diluted in a solution of propylene glycol.

These electronic cigarettes first caught the attention of the Chinese people in 2004, when it was first commercially distributed in China. This was courtesy of Hon Lik's company, "Ru Yan", which roughly translates to "Resembling Smoking". Their products were first imported in 2005 and they received their first international patent in 2007.

In 2006, Tariq Sheikh invented an even more modernized version of the electronic cigarette, called the "Cartomizer". This version incorporated the heating coil into the liquid chamber. It was first distributed to the public in the United Kingdom, in

Chapter 1:

History and Brief Introduction

Sometimes referred to as an electronic vaping device, electronic nicotine delivery system, or personal vaporizer, the E-Cigarette is a battery-powered device you can use to smoke. Due to a heating element within the device, the electronic cigarette can vaporize a liquid solution. These liquid solutions contain a wide variety of flavors, depending on the smoker's preference. To appeal to cigarette smokers, some liquid flavorings contain nicotine. However, there are still nicotine free options.

The history of electronic cigarettes dates back to 1963, when Herbert B. Gilbert patented something he described as a "non-tobacco smokeless cigarette". This smokeless cigarette was said to have been able to replace burning paper and tobacco with moist, heated, flavored air. Although Gilbert's invention was accepted by a couple of companies during the next few years, it never really materialized into a large-scale movement and was still not

Whether you plan to switch over from traditional cigarettes, start with electronic cigarettes, or just want to know more about why this trend is becoming so popular, it is important to know all the benefits and risks involved.

It is recommend to take notes while reading the book. This will ensure you get the most out of the information in here. The notes will help you to pinpoint exactly what you need to look for.

Lastly, it is encouraged for you to do your own research on specifics you want to look deeper into. The more you understand about electronic cigarettes, the more educated your decision-making process will be when purchasing different parts or giving advice to   others.

Introduction

This short book is for people interested in learning more about electronic cigarettes and not sure where to start or what information to rely on. It was created in response to the high demand of people wanting to know more about electronic cigarettes and why they are the wave of the future.

Today, the Internet has many articles and misinformation about electronic cigarettes that confuse people interested in learning about this revolutionary craze and possibly interested in purchasing an electronic cigarette of their own.

This will be a short, concise guide for everything you need to know before getting started. Understanding the history of these products and the current innovations in the market is key to predicting what the future will hold. We will also go over the different variables and options a person has in purchasing their own electronic cigarette device.

Table of Contents

presentation of the information is without contract or any type of guarantee assurance.

The trademarks that are used are without any consent, and the publication of the trademark is without permission or backing by the trademark owner. All trademarks and brands within this book are for clarifying purposes only and are the owned by the owners themselves, not affiliated with this document.

electronic cigarettes in public spaces or private establishments.

Voltage, or Power Vaporizers, have an electronic chip that allows users to control their vaping usage. Because of this type of vaporizer, you would no longer have to replace the atomizers with lower or higher electric resistance to get them to work. These can save you time and energy if you are interested.

Mechanical Vaporizers, meanwhile, are non-electric devices and are activated via spring or magnetic mechanisms. They are solder-free and rely entirely on the power of the battery. Using vaporizers such as this will lower the risk of battery explosions because they have little power.

From 50,000 users in 2008, the number of electronic cigarette users, also known as "vapers", has grown to around 3.2 million in 2012. "Vape meets" are social gatherings for electronic cigarette users and are common in most stores that sell electronic cigarettes. These events are also sometimes held in bars or pubs.

Aside from being deemed safer than traditional cigarettes, some people enjoy electronic cigarettes as a hobby. These hobbyists collect electronic cigarette devices, known as APVs, not because they are economical or easy to use, but because they are unique and shaped differently. These APVs are usually stored as a collection and are often for display only, or they may just be used occasionally.

There is no smell of tobacco or burnt products when you use electronic cigarettes. Again, it only contains vapor, flavorings, and the amount of nicotine you choose. You can also choose not to add any nicotine if you only want to taste the flavor.

Many organizations have urged the government to require electronic cigarette manufacturers to test their products for safety before releasing them to the market. Again, this will be an on-going topic, as using electronic cigarettes is becoming more common.

In 2012, Imperial Tobacco, a British multi-national company, bought the intellectual property rights of Hon Lik's invention for $75 million. This was so they could reproduce and manufacture more electronic cigarettes and distribute them throughout the country and possibly export them worldwide.

Lastly, even though electronic cigarettes are safer than traditional cigarettes by many standards, it is ultimately up to you to choose whether you want to stop smoking altogether, with or without the help of electronic cigarettes. If your top concern is health, it is probably best to avoid ingesting chemicals altogether.

Chapter 6:

How to Choose an E-Cigarette

Different strokes for different folks. This saying is especially applicable to vapers. Due to the advancement in e-cig technology, many types of vape machines have appeared on the market. Because of that, preferences have developed.

And to be honest, the same reason has made a mess. Elitism arose, and new vape users have become confused on what to buy and use. Will it be minis? Will it be a telescope? Should you go for a full mech?

If you are an aspiring vaper, then this might have become a dilemma for you. You visit the Web and see that people do not agree on one type. And if you ask somebody you know, he/she might give a different answer.

APVs and Mods

Let us start with possibly the most popular type of e-cig — APV (Advanced Personal Vaporizers) or most popularly known as mods. It has been explained in the earlier parts of this book, but what exactly are mods?

Mods technically came from the word "modifications". As manufacturers could create and verify, there is little harm in using vapes — as long as they are used properly — they gave vapers the opportunity to create their own customized vapes.

Mods surfaced when community DIYers started experimenting with their own customized e-cigs. Different batteries were used. Different wicking methods were developed. The development was too fast, and the community was too passionate about it, so it got to the point that some have developed insane setups.

APVs give the most freedom one can have when using a vape. The biggest downsides with mods are the risks involved and performance. A user who is unknowledgeable of how the battery works — or how electricity works — will concoct his own recipe for disaster if he goes for mods and becomes addicted to modifying his equipment.

Because of that, get a mod at your own risk. But whatever your reason is for getting into vaping, as long as it is not to make clouds, then any other type of e-cig will work for you.

Anyway, in the most basic sense, mods are cases where you can just put in a battery you want to use, install an atomizer of your choice, and put all the bells and whistles you want in it. Most manufacturers sell complete sets of mods, and users can just remove and replace some of its parts.

And due to it giving you freedom to customize, you can achieve a high-performing vape. If you have seen cloud makers, they are using mods.

Anyway, APVs have three sub-types. The risk, performance, safety, price, and flexibility all vary depending on the sub-type.

.

Electronic Mod

The electronic mod is the type that commonly comes with the bells and whistles. However, it can be said, if you want to have definite control of your vape, and you prioritize safety, then an electronic mod is for you.

Electronic mods typically come with some basic circuitry that can regulate the electricity that goes around the battery and the atomizers. A common feature of this circuitry is an auto shutoff feature when the voltage of the vape is going over the set threshold or if the vape's temperature is also going over the threshold.

To give you full control over your vape, some electronic mods come with small LCD screens that give crucial information about your battery and even the amount of juice that you have left. Aside from that, you can use that screen as a control panel to control the voltage that you want to flow, as well as other unique configurations.

The biggest disadvantage is that electronic mods can be the most expensive e-cig out there. Also, weight will be a definite factor you want to consider. Due to the added electronics or other features, electronic mods are often heavier than contemporary sub-types.

Mechanical Mod

This type is the most basic vape you can find in the market. The mechanical mod does not come with any additional features. Usually, it is just an empty case of stainless steel tube, where you can put a battery and place an atomizer on top.

It involves no type of wire, except for the kanthal wire on the atomizer. There is no solder. It is basically a metal tube (some mechanical mods use the common box type design).

Possibly, this is the toughest e-cig to build on the market. With no circuitry or delicate wirings, you will not have to worry too much when you drop it or place it in a cramped place, like your pocket. Despite that, it is not advised that you to situate a mechanical mod in cramped places or attempt to drop it.

Also, it can be argued that most mechanical or full mechanical mods are lightweight. And because it has no intricate wiring or circuitry, it is often cheaper than its electronic counterpart. Safety-wise, mechanical mods have no built-in safety mechanism.

For a new user, I will emphasize this to you: Do not get a mechanical mod for your first vape. The risk of it suddenly catching fire is high. If the button for the vape gets pressed for a long time, there is no circuitry that will save it from overheating and over-discharging. With no knowledge regarding the battery and how electric resistance works, you will only get into an accident with it.

Needless to say, there are ways to make it work "a bit safer". And those methods will have their own chapter, since they are also applicable to other e-cig types.

Basic Electrical Mod

The basic electrical mod is also the mod that was developed first. It is an electronic mod with the basic safety features. It is relatively cheaper, and most people recommend newbies to get the basic electrical mod first when going with the mod route.

Mini

Mini is the first e-cigarette that started the commercial growth of the vaping industry. Minis are shaped like a real cigarette. Most models work pneumatically. It means you need not press a button to vape. Just inhale through the mini, and it will automatically turn on and produce vapor.

Aside from that, minis have LED indicators that let you know if it is operating. It is often on the other end. Because of that light, it will appear like you are using a real cigarette, since the LED light looks like a cigarette's glowing ember.

Compared to mods, minis are lightweight, discreet, and small. Most people recommend newbies to start with minis. If you are looking for specific reliable makes and models, you can choose from KR8 (or KR808), M401, 901, and 510.

It has its own advantages and disadvantages. Aside from its key features that allow easy transition for smokers to start vaping, minis are relatively cheaper than mods. Minis are composed of simple small parts to make it work, which make it easier to produce and sell for a cheaper price.

If you are a light smoker, feel no need to make big clouds of smoke, and just want to try vaping, a mini might be the right equipment for you. But if you smoke a lot and foresee that you will get "addicted" to vaping, then expect to smoke a lot less when you buy a mini.

When it comes to disadvantages, minis have a lot. First off, they have short battery life. After a few puffs on a mini, it will be drained. Frequent recharging of the device is needed (although this can be a huge plus to light smokers, since it will truly emulate a cigarette).

To compensate for this, you can buy multiple minis. It will cost more, but the total expense is low enough to compare to getting a decent mod. Having multiple minis will extend the time you can vape outside.

Second, they are disposable and fragile. The circuitry within minis is not that complex; however, its connections are connected using thin brittle wires. Just one drop can make those wires disconnect and render it useless. Why the low quality materials and craftsmanship? Well, they are disposable. Only a few select brands create sturdy minis.

Third, it can be messy to use. Unlike mods, minis use cartridges to deliver their juice to the minis' atomizers. The cartridge is the "butt" of the mini. Inside that cartridge is a small plastic container, where the juice is located. On its end is an aluminum/plastic covering. When you insert the cartridge to the mini, the pointed shape of the atomizer will puncture it to allow the juice to flow into the atomizer.

Unfortunately, that method of juice delivery is not leak-proof. Since there is a hole in the cartridge where the vapor comes out, the juice could easily leak there when the mini is placed upside down. Mods have the same structure, but the juice is often bound to wicks, so no juice is flowing around modern atomizers.

Fourth, you do not have full control of the flavor of your mini. Creating your own cartridges is troublesome, and you will be stuck with what manufacturers provide. This is a small issue, but if you get into vaping, this could potentially become a notable drawback.

Fifth, the cartridges are disposable. The expense of purchasing a lot of cartridges might be small at first, but it will add up if you become a habitual vaper.

Sixth, the amount of vapor you inhale will be too limited for some people. Minis have a built-in limiter to prevent them from overheating.

eGo or the Mid-Size Type

After the popularity of minis arose, the mid-size type or eGo models were created and introduced to the market. The eGo type solves most issues the mini has, but at a few expenses. The mid-size type has longer battery life, greater juice capacity, and durability. However, in exchange for those feature improvements, mid-size vapes are longer, heavier, and thicker than minis. Nevertheless, they are thinner and lighter than mods.

The main reason mid-size e-cigs could improve performance, but became heavier, is batteries. You may have realized by now that batteries are the deciding factor for a vape's performance.

As of now, eGo vapes are the most widely used vapes. This is mostly due to eGo being enough to provide the exact performance for most people. The batteries within eGo models can last a day without charging for a regular vaper.

Also, most mid-size models come with clearomizers. With a clearomizer, you need not drip or change cartridges if you have enough juice in your tank. In addition, with a clearomizer, you can see how much juice you still have in your e-cig.

Another feature that comes with eGo types is a battery controller. Just like minis, eGo has circuits to prevent over-heating. And some come with voltage controllers, which can allow you to modify the performance of your e-cig.

Briefly, mid-size e-cigs are more like a basic and weaker electronic mod. That can be helped, since eGo e-cigs were the precursors to modding and the creation of mods.

All right, everything sounds great regarding mid-size, right? Yes. To be frank, this is the basic and standard vape most people have. If you fear the disadvantages of minis and you think mods are too much for you to handle, then it is better for you to settle with eGo or mid-size.

But wait... There is also a potential problem with eGo. Due to its popularity, it has been the center of duplication and massive production of cheap clones. Yep. Clones.

There is nothing wrong with duplicates or clones. The biggest problem is that most clones' quality is sub-par. Sub-par may not even be the right term - but more like crappy and dangerous. It is highly recommended that you make sure you only buy from trusted manufacturers.

Clone makers have gone too low to spread substandard products that can easily cause fire and explosion incidents. Sure, you can vape with those eGo clones. You can prevent accidents by being extra careful. But being too careful still may not be enough.

By now, the number of fire and explosion accidents related to vaping is tremendously high. And it is almost overwhelmingly caused by cheap clones. If you want to know more about how many people experience accidents with cheap clones, you can just go over to Reddit and ECF (E-Cigarette Forum).

Chapter 7:

Safety Guidelines

If you are switching to vaping to save yourself from smoking, it would be ironic if you hurt yourself because of fire, explosion, and poisoning by not following any safety guidelines. Let us be honest here: Vaping is not 100% safe.

Most vapers will agree, and some will defend it as safe to use a modern vape. However, at the end of the day, you are putting a stick of battery you are short-circuiting near your mouth. The risk is big. A lit stick of cigarette can only burn a small patch of skin. But a battery on fire or explosion will be too much for a regular Band-Aid to handle.

So, to prevent that scenario, please read and follow the safety guidelines below. To be frank, if this guideline was detailed, this chapter would be as long as all the previous chapters combined. But do not be discouraged. To be honest, they are simple steps to ensure your safety. Do them once, and they can become second nature to you when you vape.

Always Be Mindful of the Amount of Juice in Your E-Cig

Seems simple enough. If you are using a clearomizer, this would be an easy task. If you are using a cartomizer or a simple drip type atomizer, then it will need practice.

Always check the e-liquid in your clearomizer. If it is already down to the the last few drips, then refill it. Do not wait until you empty your tank. If you are planning to change the flavor of your liquid, then wait for it to be empty. But it will be much better to just throw out the remaining liquid instead.

What will happen if you do not do this and you run out of juice? First, you will inhale smoke from a burnt wick or atomizer. Second, your wick might get burnt. If that happens, the flavor of any e-liquid you will put in will be compromised and smell burnt. When that happens, replace your wick immediately.

Third, letting your atomizer produce dry heat for a long time can ruin it. And once it gets hot, you are risking your battery.

Fourth, this scenario will produce low amounts of vapor, so there is no point in emptying your liquid in your   e-cig   to   the   last   drop.

Let Your E-Cig Breathe for A While

Atomizers, whatever type, can get burning hot if used non-stop for a few minutes. If you do not want your fingers to get scalded, let it breathe for a while. Also, you must breathe yourself. Do not be too greedy with the vape. If you have a spare atomizer, it would be a good idea to switch between them when one gets hot.

Be Cautious When Charging

The first rule in the game is that you must never charge while you sleep or let the charger be left unattended. One of the major reasons vaping accidents happen is careless battery charging. Also, make sure you follow the manual that comes with your vape and charger.

This is not just for charging electronic cigarettes. This goes for any electronic device you charge. If you leave your batteries or devices unattended while charging, they might overcharge. And when overcharged, a battery can get hot and explode or start a fire. Always make it a habit to remove your battery or device from the charger once it is charged.

Also, do not leave your batteries on top of flammable surfaces or items, like carpets.

Use The Charger That Comes with Your Battery or E-Cig

When it comes to electronics, you can never be too cautious. Always use the charger supplied with your e-cig or battery. Do not mix and match chargers, especially if you do not understand polarity, voltage rating, and amperage. Also, if you need a replacement, always get one from a trusted manufacturer or supplier.

Be Cognizant of Where You Leave Your Batteries and E-Cigs

Never leave your batteries and e-cig in a place that's exposed to direct sunlight. Also, never leave it in places that are extremely cold or hot. Your batteries should always be at room temperature. Ideally, most batteries, especial Li-ion (Lithium-Ion) batteries, should be in a place with a temperature of 15 degrees Celsius (59 degrees Fahrenheit).

If you will not use the batteries for some time, make sure you store them half-charged. Charge your e-cig first, use it for a while, and then store.

If you are going to store your e-cig, cover the mouthpiece with a small plastic or paper tip to prevent your juice from evaporating. Juice left exposed to open air will taste bland and weak. Also, be sure your e-cig's button is locked.

Make Sure to Carry Your E-Cig with Care

Do not just put your e-cig in your pocket. As much as possible, bring your e-cig bag with you. All of your e-cig paraphernalia should be well separated from each other. Also, your bag must be lint and dust-free. You would not want those elements to enter your atomizer. In addition, turn it off or lock the button. Another commonly used protocol is to separate the batteries from your e-cig if you have a mod.

Being careless with this part might lead to an accidental short circuit. And the last thing you want to happen is a fire or explosion near your crotch. However, remove all the coins, keys, or other metallic stuff from your pocket to prevent an accident if you badly need to put it there and do not have your bag with you.

The same goes for your batteries. Never lump them with coins and other metallic trinkets.

Do Not Create E-Juice of Your Own Without Any Decent Knowledge

One can become a connoisseur of e-juices after vaping for some time. And some people want to achieve a flavor that will truly suit their taste buds. This leads to mixing DIY e-juices.

As a piece of advice, never think of making your e-juice first, especially if you are planning to make ones that contain nicotine. Nicotine in its purest liquid form is toxic. Just one wrong move can poison you. Some extracts or flavorings might contain ingredients or elements not suitable for vaping.

Two are alcohol and oil. Vaping a juice with those in it can result in dizziness. If you know what you are doing, then those two can be controlled. And unfortunately, they are just two things of many you should watch out for.

It should go without saying, but you should be smart enough not to drink e-juice, especially ones with nicotine content. A few drops can easily ruin your stomach. But if it accidentally gets into your mouth, quickly spit and rinse your mouth with a mouthwash or water.

Yet, despite the warning, some of you will venture to taste it. Yes, it tastes pleasant — mildly sweet and bitter if it has nicotine. Because of that, make sure you also keep your e-cig and e-juice away from children.

If the juice with nicotine gets on your skin, wipe it fast. Skin absorbs nicotine. And if it is pure nicotine spilled on you, you better prepare yourself, since you might need to visit a doctor. You can easily get nicotine poisoning from that incident alone.

Health Condition and Allergy-Related Issues

Before you start vaping, make sure you are not allergic to the contents of an e-juice. What are the ingredients in an e-juice, anyway? Primarily, it comprises glycerin. It could be vegetable glycerin (VG), propylene glycol (PG), or both. These create the vapor. Depending on the ratio between them, your e-cig's vapor can come out thick, sweet, thin, or strong.

The second primary component in an e-juice is the flavoring. Most DIY e-juice makers use flavorings and extracts for baking. Depending on the extract, the juice might come with little quantities of alcohol, oil, and preservatives. Always check the label on the e-juice bottle.

The third component, which is also optional, is nicotine. E-juices often come with a label on how much nicotine is added. If you do not want to vape nicotine, you can opt for one with zero nicotine content.

Propylene glycol is the main ingredient responsible for what they call "throat hit". Throat hit is a term used to describe the sensation of having warm smoke hitting your throat when smoking. Since vapor from e-cigs are not that hot, propylene glycol is needed to emulate that sensation.

If you cough after a hit from an e-cig, the PG in your e-juice can be the reason. One way to solve this is to get an e-juice with less PG concentration or have a flavor with menthol in it.

Aside from providing throat hit, too much PG can cause itchy eyes, headaches, nausea, swelling, rashes, hives, headaches, wheezing, and sore throat. Most of the time, all new vapers experience these symptoms/effects. It will usually be gone after a week or two of vaping.

However, if all or any persists, contact your doctor. Or you can just switch to a juice with a better VG/PG ratio for you.

Conclusion

Hopefully this short book helped you learn more about electronic cigarettes, what they are made of, the different options you have, and the positive and negative aspects of using them. Now that you have learned the important factors regarding electronic cigarettes, you can finally decide if you want to use one or if you would recommend them to your family and friends.

Plus, the addition to your knowledge base doesn't hurt, right? It's good to know about new innovations, because it keeps you in the know, especially in a world where every big city has electronic cigarette shops sprouting up on a monthly basis.

The next step is to share what you have learned with other people, especially those who have been vaping for a while or who would like to try an electronic cigarette for the first time. You should share with them what you have learned, especially the negative aspects of using electronic cigarettes, because it is essential to keep track of one's health and not get lost in a fad to impress other people.

Be sure to make responsible decisions and always consult with your doctor! Thank you and good luck in your own journey!

www.ingramcontent.com/pod-product-compliance
Lightning Source LLC
Chambersburg PA
CBHW070949180526
45168CB00003B/1179